blessed af

THIS JOURNAL BELONGS TO:

_____

How about a freebie?

Email books@bluetruckbooks.com, tell us something you are thankful for, and we'll send something fun your way!

Blessed AF: A Gratitude Journal
Copyright © 2020 by BlueTruck Books
First Edition, April 2020

Blue Truck BOOKS

Published by:
BlueTruck Books
1218 Country Rd
Franklin, TN 37069

All rights reserved. Blessed AF: A Gratitude Journal is under copyright protection. No part of this book may be used or reproduced in any manner whatsoever without written permission except in the case of brief quotations embodied in critcal articles and reviews.

Compiled by Vienna Rovenstine
Designed by Emily Hume
Typeset by Emily Hume / emilykayhdesigns@gmail.com
ISBN: 978-1-7346712-0-9
*Special thanks to Greg Boyd of Woodland Hills church and the inspiration for the happy pill. For more excellent insights on gratitude and life, check it out: https:whchurch.org

Before you get started...

Have you ever met a person who said they did not want to be more happy?
Here is some really good news. In multiple clinical studies, researchers found that the common denominator for happy people is...gratitude.

Just a few of the benefits people reported after 30 day clinical trials:
- Happiness levels increased
- Less anxiety and worry
- Better and more restful sleep
- Started exercising (without being prompted)
- More social connections and empathy

...and that is why we have created this gratitude journal. It's a safe place to capture and record those things you are truly blessed with. Think of it as your daily happy pill.

Enjoy!

blessed af

JAN FEB MAR APR MAY JUN JUL AUG SEP OCT NOV DEC
1 2 3 4 5 6 7 8 9 10 11 12 13 14 15 16 17 18 19 20 21 22 23 24 25 26 27 28 29 30 31

SOMETHING GOOD THAT HAPPENED TODAY
___
___
___
___

SOMEONE OR SOMETHING I AM THANKFUL FOR AND WHY
___
___
___
___

MY GOOD DEED, HAPPY THOUGHT, OR KIND ACT FOR THE DAY
___
___
___
___

Nothing is impossible, the word itself says "I'm possible!"
- Audrey Hepburn

blessed af

JAN FEB MAR APR MAY JUN JUL AUG SEP OCT NOV DEC
1 2 3 4 5 6 7 8 9 10 11 12 13 14 15 16 17 18 19 20 21 22 23 24 25 26 27 28 29 30 31

SOMETHING GOOD THAT HAPPENED TODAY
_____
_____
_____
_____

SOMEONE OR SOMETHING I AM THANKFUL FOR AND WHY
_____
_____
_____
_____

MY GOOD DEED, HAPPY THOUGHT, OR KIND ACT FOR THE DAY
_____
_____
_____
_____

Your voice is a gift. Enjoy it and share it.
- Hannah Ann Sluss

blessed af

JAN FEB MAR APR MAY JUN JUL AUG SEP OCT NOV DEC
1 2 3 4 5 6 7 8 9 10 11 12 13 14 15 16 17 18 19 20 21 22 23 24 25 26 27 28 29 30 31

SOMETHING GOOD THAT HAPPENED TODAY

_____
_____
_____
_____

SOMEONE OR SOMETHING I AM THANKFUL FOR AND WHY

_____
_____
_____
_____

MY GOOD DEED, HAPPY THOUGHT, OR KIND ACT FOR THE DAY

_____
_____
_____
_____

Spread love everywhere you go. Let no one ever come to you without leaving happier.
- Mother Teresa

blessed af

JAN FEB MAR APR MAY JUN JUL AUG SEP OCT NOV DEC
1   2   3   4   5   6   7   8   9   10   11   12   13   14   15   16   17   18   19   20   21   22   23   24   25   26   27   28   29   30   31

SOMETHING GOOD THAT HAPPENED TODAY
_____
_____
_____
_____

SOMEONE OR SOMETHING I AM THANKFUL
FOR AND WHY
_____
_____
_____
_____

MY GOOD DEED, HAPPY THOUGHT, OR
KIND ACT FOR THE DAY
_____
_____
_____
_____

> **What separates privilege from entitlement is gratitude.**
> - Brene Brown

blessed af

JAN FEB MAR APR MAY JUN JUL AUG SEP OCT NOV DEC
1 2 3 4 5 6 7 8 9 10 11 12 13 14 15 16 17 18 19 20 21 22 23 24 25 26 27 28 29 30 31

SOMETHING GOOD THAT HAPPENED TODAY
___
___
___
___

SOMEONE OR SOMETHING I AM THANKFUL FOR AND WHY
___
___
___
___

MY GOOD DEED, HAPPY THOUGHT, OR KIND ACT FOR THE DAY
___
___
___
___

**If you obey all the rules, you miss all the fun.
- Katharine Hepburn**

blessed af

| JAN | FEB | MAR | APR | MAY | JUN | JUL | AUG | SEP | OCT | NOV | DEC |

1 2 3 4 5 6 7 8 9 10 11 12 13 14 15 16 17 18 19 20 21 22 23 24 25 26 27 28 29 30 31

SOMETHING GOOD THAT HAPPENED TODAY

_____
_____
_____
_____

SOMEONE OR SOMETHING I AM THANKFUL FOR AND WHY

_____
_____
_____
_____

MY GOOD DEED, HAPPY THOUGHT, OR KIND ACT FOR THE DAY

_____
_____
_____
_____

> When I started counting my blessings, my whole life turned around.
> - Willie Nelson

blessed af

JAN   FEB   MAR   APR   MAY   JUN   JUL   AUG   SEP   OCT   NOV   DEC
1 2 3 4 5 6 7 8 9 10 11 12 13 14 15 16 17 18 19 20 21 22 23 24 25 26 27 28 29 30 31

SOMETHING GOOD THAT HAPPENED TODAY
_____
_____
_____
_____

SOMEONE OR SOMETHING I AM THANKFUL FOR AND WHY
_____
_____
_____
_____

MY GOOD DEED, HAPPY THOUGHT, OR KIND ACT FOR THE DAY
_____
_____
_____
_____

**It is never too late to be what you might have been.
- George Eliot**

blessed af

JAN FEB MAR APR MAY JUN JUL AUG SEP OCT NOV DEC
1 2 3 4 5 6 7 8 9 10 11 12 13 14 15 16 17 18 19 20 21 22 23 24 25 26 27 28 29 30 31

SOMETHING GOOD THAT HAPPENED TODAY
_____
_____
_____
_____

SOMEONE OR SOMETHING I AM THANKFUL
FOR AND WHY
_____
_____
_____
_____

MY GOOD DEED, HAPPY THOUGHT, OR
KIND ACT FOR THE DAY
_____
_____
_____
_____

**Roll with the punches and enjoy
every minute of it.
- Meghan Markle**

blessed af

JAN FEB MAR APR MAY JUN JUL AUG SEP OCT NOV DEC
1 2 3 4 5 6 7 8 9 10 11 12 13 14 15 16 17 18 19 20 21 22 23 24 25 26 27 28 29 30 31

SOMETHING GOOD THAT HAPPENED TODAY

_____
_____
_____
_____

SOMEONE OR SOMETHING I AM THANKFUL FOR AND WHY

_____
_____
_____
_____

MY GOOD DEED, HAPPY THOUGHT, OR KIND ACT FOR THE DAY

_____
_____
_____
_____

Don't look at your feet to see if you are doing it right. Just dance.
- Anne Lamott

blessed af

JAN FEB MAR APR MAY JUN JUL AUG SEP OCT NOV DEC
1 2 3 4 5 6 7 8 9 10 11 12 13 14 15 16 17 18 19 20 21 22 23 24 25 26 27 28 29 30 31

SOMETHING GOOD THAT HAPPENED TODAY
_____
_____
_____
_____

SOMEONE OR SOMETHING I AM THANKFUL FOR AND WHY
_____
_____
_____
_____

MY GOOD DEED, HAPPY THOUGHT, OR KIND ACT FOR THE DAY
_____
_____
_____
_____

> I've learned that making a living is
> not the same thing as making a life.
> - Maya Angelou

blessed af

JAN FEB MAR APR MAY JUN JUL AUG SEP OCT NOV DEC
1 2 3 4 5 6 7 8 9 10 11 12 13 14 15 16 17 18 19 20 21 22 23 24 25 26 27 28 29 30 31

SOMETHING GOOD THAT HAPPENED TODAY

___

SOMEONE OR SOMETHING I AM THANKFUL FOR AND WHY

___

MY GOOD DEED, HAPPY THOUGHT, OR KIND ACT FOR THE DAY

___

If you're offered a seat on a rocket ship, don't ask what seat! Just get on.
- Sheryl Sandberg

blessed af

JAN FEB MAR APR MAY JUN JUL AUG SEP OCT NOV DEC
1 2 3 4 5 6 7 8 9 10 11 12 13 14 15 16 17 18 19 20 21 22 23 24 25 26 27 28 29 30 31

SOMETHING GOOD THAT HAPPENED TODAY
_____
_____
_____
_____

SOMEONE OR SOMETHING I AM THANKFUL FOR AND WHY
_____
_____
_____
_____

MY GOOD DEED, HAPPY THOUGHT, OR KIND ACT FOR THE DAY
_____
_____
_____
_____

> Love yourself first, and everything else falls into line. You really have to love yourself to get anything done in this world.
> - Lucille Ball

blessed af

JAN FEB MAR APR MAY JUN JUL AUG SEP OCT NOV DEC
1 2 3 4 5 6 7 8 9 10 11 12 13 14 15 16 17 18 19 20 21 22 23 24 25 26 27 28 29 30 31

SOMETHING GOOD THAT HAPPENED TODAY
___
___
___
___

SOMEONE OR SOMETHING I AM THANKFUL FOR AND WHY
___
___
___
___

MY GOOD DEED, HAPPY THOUGHT, OR KIND ACT FOR THE DAY
___
___
___
___

Learn from the mistakes of others. You can't live long enough to make them all yourself.
- Eleanor Roosevelt

blessed af

JAN FEB MAR APR MAY JUN JUL AUG SEP OCT NOV DEC
1 2 3 4 5 6 7 8 9 10 11 12 13 14 15 16 17 18 19 20 21 22 23 24 25 26 27 28 29 30 31

SOMETHING GOOD THAT HAPPENED TODAY

_____
_____
_____
_____

SOMEONE OR SOMETHING I AM THANKFUL FOR AND WHY

_____
_____
_____
_____

MY GOOD DEED, HAPPY THOUGHT, OR KIND ACT FOR THE DAY

_____
_____
_____
_____

The question isn't who is going to let me, it's who is going to stop me.
- Ayn Rand

blessed af

JAN FEB MAR APR MAY JUN JUL AUG SEP OCT NOV DEC
1 2 3 4 5 6 7 8 9 10 11 12 13 14 15 16 17 18 19 20 21 22 23 24 25 26 27 28 29 30 31

SOMETHING GOOD THAT HAPPENED TODAY

_____
_____
_____
_____

SOMEONE OR SOMETHING I AM THANKFUL FOR AND WHY

_____
_____
_____
_____

MY GOOD DEED, HAPPY THOUGHT, OR KIND ACT FOR THE DAY

_____
_____
_____
_____

It's one of the greatest gifts you can give yourself, to forgive. Forgive everybody.
- Maya Angelou

blessed af

JAN FEB MAR APR MAY JUN JUL AUG SEP OCT NOV DEC
1 2 3 4 5 6 7 8 9 10 11 12 13 14 15 16 17 18 19 20 21 22 23 24 25 26 27 28 29 30 31

SOMETHING GOOD THAT HAPPENED TODAY
_____
_____
_____
_____

SOMEONE OR SOMETHING I AM THANKFUL FOR AND WHY
_____
_____
_____
_____

MY GOOD DEED, HAPPY THOUGHT, OR KIND ACT FOR THE DAY
_____
_____
_____
_____

I didn't get there by wishing for it or hoping for it, but by working for it.
- Estée Lauder

blessed af

JAN FEB MAR APR MAY JUN JUL AUG SEP OCT NOV DEC
1 2 3 4 5 6 7 8 9 10 11 12 13 14 15 16 17 18 19 20 21 22 23 24 25 26 27 28 29 30 31

SOMETHING GOOD THAT HAPPENED TODAY
_____
_____
_____
_____

SOMEONE OR SOMETHING I AM THANKFUL FOR AND WHY
_____
_____
_____
_____

MY GOOD DEED, HAPPY THOUGHT, OR KIND ACT FOR THE DAY
_____
_____
_____
_____

Aerodynamically the bumblebee shouldn't be able to fly, but the bumblebee doesn't know that so it goes on flying anyway.
- Mary Kay Ash

blessed af

JAN FEB MAR APR MAY JUN JUL AUG SEP OCT NOV DEC
1 2 3 4 5 6 7 8 9 10 11 12 13 14 15 16 17 18 19 20 21 22 23 24 25 26 27 28 29 30 31

SOMETHING GOOD THAT HAPPENED TODAY
_____
_____
_____
_____

SOMEONE OR SOMETHING I AM THANKFUL FOR AND WHY
_____
_____
_____
_____

MY GOOD DEED, HAPPY THOUGHT, OR KIND ACT FOR THE DAY
_____
_____
_____
_____

Gratitude helps you to grow and expand; gratitude brings joy and laughter into your life and into the lives of all those around you.
- Eileen Caddy

blessed af

JAN FEB MAR APR MAY JUN JUL AUG SEP OCT NOV DEC
1 2 3 4 5 6 7 8 9 10 11 12 13 14 15 16 17 18 19 20 21 22 23 24 25 26 27 28 29 30 31

SOMETHING GOOD THAT HAPPENED TODAY

_____
_____
_____
_____

SOMEONE OR SOMETHING I AM THANKFUL FOR AND WHY

_____
_____
_____
_____

MY GOOD DEED, HAPPY THOUGHT, OR KIND ACT FOR THE DAY

_____
_____
_____
_____

The difference between successful people and others is how long they spend time feeling sorry for themselves.
- Barbara Corcoran

blessed af

JAN   FEB   MAR   APR   MAY   JUN   JUL   AUG   SEP   OCT   NOV   DEC
1 2 3 4 5 6 7 8 9 10 11 12 13 14 15 16 17 18 19 20 21 22 23 24 25 26 27 28 29 30 31

SOMETHING GOOD THAT HAPPENED TODAY
_____
_____
_____
_____

SOMEONE OR SOMETHING I AM THANKFUL FOR AND WHY
_____
_____
_____
_____

MY GOOD DEED, HAPPY THOUGHT, OR KIND ACT FOR THE DAY
_____
_____
_____
_____

> When you embrace your difference, your DNA, your look or heritage or religion or your unusual name, that's when you start to shine.
> - Bethenny Frankel

blessed af

JAN FEB MAR APR MAY JUN JUL AUG SEP OCT NOV DEC
1 2 3 4 5 6 7 8 9 10 11 12 13 14 15 16 17 18 19 20 21 22 23 24 25 26 27 28 29 30 31

SOMETHING GOOD THAT HAPPENED TODAY

_____
_____
_____
_____

SOMEONE OR SOMETHING I AM THANKFUL FOR AND WHY

_____
_____
_____
_____

MY GOOD DEED, HAPPY THOUGHT, OR KIND ACT FOR THE DAY

_____
_____
_____
_____

Be a first-rate version of yourself, instead of a second-rate version of somebody else.
- Judy Garland

blessed af

JAN FEB MAR APR MAY JUN JUL AUG SEP OCT NOV DEC
1 2 3 4 5 6 7 8 9 10 11 12 13 14 15 16 17 18 19 20 21 22 23 24 25 26 27 28 29 30 31

SOMETHING GOOD THAT HAPPENED TODAY
___
___
___
___

SOMEONE OR SOMETHING I AM THANKFUL FOR AND WHY
___
___
___
___

MY GOOD DEED, HAPPY THOUGHT, OR KIND ACT FOR THE DAY
___
___
___
___

He is a wise man who does not grieve for the things which he has not, but rejoices for those which he has.
- Epictetus

blessed af

JAN FEB MAR APR MAY JUN JUL AUG SEP OCT NOV DEC
1 2 3 4 5 6 7 8 9 10 11 12 13 14 15 16 17 18 19 20 21 22 23 24 25 26 27 28 29 30 31

SOMETHING GOOD THAT HAPPENED TODAY
___
___
___
___

SOMEONE OR SOMETHING I AM THANKFUL FOR AND WHY
___
___
___
___

MY GOOD DEED, HAPPY THOUGHT, OR KIND ACT FOR THE DAY
___
___
___
___

When one's mind is made up, this diminishes fear; knowing what must be done does away with fear.
- Rosa Parks

blessed af

JAN FEB MAR APR MAY JUN JUL AUG SEP OCT NOV DEC
1 2 3 4 5 6 7 8 9 10 11 12 13 14 15 16 17 18 19 20 21 22 23 24 25 26 27 28 29 30 31

SOMETHING GOOD THAT HAPPENED TODAY
_____
_____
_____
_____

SOMEONE OR SOMETHING I AM THANKFUL FOR AND WHY
_____
_____
_____
_____

MY GOOD DEED, HAPPY THOUGHT, OR KIND ACT FOR THE DAY
_____
_____
_____
_____

> It is better to light a candle than curse the darkness.
> - Eleanor Roosevelt

blessed af

JAN FEB MAR APR MAY JUN JUL AUG SEP OCT NOV DEC
1 2 3 4 5 6 7 8 9 10 11 12 13 14 15 16 17 18 19 20 21 22 23 24 25 26 27 28 29 30 31

SOMETHING GOOD THAT HAPPENED TODAY

_____
_____
_____
_____

SOMEONE OR SOMETHING I AM THANKFUL FOR AND WHY

_____
_____
_____
_____

MY GOOD DEED, HAPPY THOUGHT, OR KIND ACT FOR THE DAY

_____
_____
_____
_____

I choose to make the rest of my life the best of my life.
- Louise Hay

blessed af

JAN FEB MAR APR MAY JUN JUL AUG SEP OCT NOV DEC
1 2 3 4 5 6 7 8 9 10 11 12 13 14 15 16 17 18 19 20 21 22 23 24 25 26 27 28 29 30 31

SOMETHING GOOD THAT HAPPENED TODAY
_____
_____
_____
_____

SOMEONE OR SOMETHING I AM THANKFUL FOR AND WHY
_____
_____
_____
_____

MY GOOD DEED, HAPPY THOUGHT, OR KIND ACT FOR THE DAY
_____
_____
_____
_____

**Done is better than perfect.
- Sheryl Sandberg**

blessed af

JAN FEB MAR APR MAY JUN JUL AUG SEP OCT NOV DEC
1 2 3 4 5 6 7 8 9 10 11 12 13 14 15 16 17 18 19 20 21 22 23 24 25 26 27 28 29 30 31

SOMETHING GOOD THAT HAPPENED TODAY

_____
_____
_____
_____
_____

SOMEONE OR SOMETHING I AM THANKFUL FOR AND WHY

_____
_____
_____
_____
_____

MY GOOD DEED, HAPPY THOUGHT, OR KIND ACT FOR THE DAY

_____
_____
_____
_____
_____

> There is no greater gift you can give or receive than to honor your calling. It's why you were born.
> - Oprah Winfrey

blessed af

JAN FEB MAR APR MAY JUN JUL AUG SEP OCT NOV DEC
1 2 3 4 5 6 7 8 9 10 11 12 13 14 15 16 17 18 19 20 21 22 23 24 25 26 27 28 29 30 31

SOMETHING GOOD THAT HAPPENED TODAY
_____
_____
_____
_____

SOMEONE OR SOMETHING I AM THANKFUL FOR AND WHY
_____
_____
_____
_____

MY GOOD DEED, HAPPY THOUGHT, OR KIND ACT FOR THE DAY
_____
_____
_____
_____

Gratitude is not only the greatest of virtues but the parent of all others.
- Marcus Tullius Cicero

blessed af

JAN FEB MAR APR MAY JUN JUL AUG SEP OCT NOV DEC
1 2 3 4 5 6 7 8 9 10 11 12 13 14 15 16 17 18 19 20 21 22 23 24 25 26 27 28 29 30 31

SOMETHING GOOD THAT HAPPENED TODAY

_____
_____
_____
_____

SOMEONE OR SOMETHING I AM THANKFUL FOR AND WHY

_____
_____
_____
_____

MY GOOD DEED, HAPPY THOUGHT, OR KIND ACT FOR THE DAY

_____
_____
_____
_____

**Every moment wasted looking back keeps us from moving forward.
- Hillary Clinton**

blessed af

JAN FEB MAR APR MAY JUN JUL AUG SEP OCT NOV DEC
1 2 3 4 5 6 7 8 9 10 11 12 13 14 15 16 17 18 19 20 21 22 23 24 25 26 27 28 29 30 31

SOMETHING GOOD THAT HAPPENED TODAY
_____
_____
_____
_____

SOMEONE OR SOMETHING I AM THANKFUL FOR AND WHY
_____
_____
_____
_____

MY GOOD DEED, HAPPY THOUGHT, OR KIND ACT FOR THE DAY
_____
_____
_____
_____

Cautious, careful people, always casting about to preserve their reputations can never effect a reform.
- Susan B. Anthony

blessed af

JAN FEB MAR APR MAY JUN JUL AUG SEP OCT NOV DEC
1 2 3 4 5 6 7 8 9 10 11 12 13 14 15 16 17 18 19 20 21 22 23 24 25 26 27 28 29 30 31

SOMETHING GOOD THAT HAPPENED TODAY
_____
_____
_____
_____

SOMEONE OR SOMETHING I AM THANKFUL FOR AND WHY
_____
_____
_____
_____

MY GOOD DEED, HAPPY THOUGHT, OR KIND ACT FOR THE DAY
_____
_____
_____
_____

**Make the most of yourself by fanning the tiny, inner sparks of possibility into flames of achievement.
- Golda Meir**

blessed af

JAN FEB MAR APR MAY JUN JUL AUG SEP OCT NOV DEC
1 2 3 4 5 6 7 8 9 10 11 12 13 14 15 16 17 18 19 20 21 22 23 24 25 26 27 28 29 30 31

SOMETHING GOOD THAT HAPPENED TODAY

_____
_____
_____
_____

SOMEONE OR SOMETHING I AM THANKFUL FOR AND WHY

_____
_____
_____
_____

MY GOOD DEED, HAPPY THOUGHT, OR KIND ACT FOR THE DAY

_____
_____
_____
_____

**If you don't like the road you're walking, start paving another one.
- Dolly Parton**

blessed af

JAN FEB MAR APR MAY JUN JUL AUG SEP OCT NOV DEC
1 2 3 4 5 6 7 8 9 10 11 12 13 14 15 16 17 18 19 20 21 22 23 24 25 26 27 28 29 30 31

SOMETHING GOOD THAT HAPPENED TODAY

_____
_____
_____
_____

SOMEONE OR SOMETHING I AM THANKFUL FOR AND WHY

_____
_____
_____
_____

MY GOOD DEED, HAPPY THOUGHT, OR KIND ACT FOR THE DAY

_____
_____
_____
_____

> **Two kinds of gratitude: The sudden kind we feel for what we take; the larger kind we feel for what we give.**
> **- Edwin Arlington Robinson**

blessed af

JAN FEB MAR APR MAY JUN JUL AUG SEP OCT NOV DEC
1 2 3 4 5 6 7 8 9 10 11 12 13 14 15 16 17 18 19 20 21 22 23 24 25 26 27 28 29 30 31

SOMETHING GOOD THAT HAPPENED TODAY
___
___
___
___

SOMEONE OR SOMETHING I AM THANKFUL FOR AND WHY
___
___
___
___

MY GOOD DEED, HAPPY THOUGHT, OR KIND ACT FOR THE DAY
___
___
___
___

No matter how difficult and painful it may be, nothing sounds as good to the soul as the truth.
- Martha Beck

blessed af

JAN FEB MAR APR MAY JUN JUL AUG SEP OCT NOV DEC
1 2 3 4 5 6 7 8 9 10 11 12 13 14 15 16 17 18 19 20 21 22 23 24 25 26 27 28 29 30 31

SOMETHING GOOD THAT HAPPENED TODAY
___
___
___

SOMEONE OR SOMETHING I AM THANKFUL FOR AND WHY
___
___
___

MY GOOD DEED, HAPPY THOUGHT, OR KIND ACT FOR THE DAY
___
___
___

**I'm not going to become anybody I don't want to become.
- Kristen Bell**

blessed af

JAN FEB MAR APR MAY JUN JUL AUG SEP OCT NOV DEC
1 2 3 4 5 6 7 8 9 10 11 12 13 14 15 16 17 18 19 20 21 22 23 24 25 26 27 28 29 30 31

SOMETHING GOOD THAT HAPPENED TODAY
_____
_____
_____
_____

SOMEONE OR SOMETHING I AM THANKFUL FOR AND WHY
_____
_____
_____
_____

MY GOOD DEED, HAPPY THOUGHT, OR KIND ACT FOR THE DAY
_____
_____
_____
_____

> Let gratitude be the pillow upon which you kneel to say your nightly prayer. And let faith be the bridge you build to overcome evil and welcome good.
> - Maya Angelou

blessed af

JAN FEB MAR APR MAY JUN JUL AUG SEP OCT NOV DEC
1 2 3 4 5 6 7 8 9 10 11 12 13 14 15 16 17 18 19 20 21 22 23 24 25 26 27 28 29 30 31

SOMETHING GOOD THAT HAPPENED TODAY
_____
_____
_____
_____

SOMEONE OR SOMETHING I AM THANKFUL FOR AND WHY
_____
_____
_____
_____

MY GOOD DEED, HAPPY THOUGHT, OR KIND ACT FOR THE DAY
_____
_____
_____
_____

In order to be irreplaceable, one must always be different.
- Coco Chanel

blessed af

JAN FEB MAR APR MAY JUN JUL AUG SEP OCT NOV DEC
1 2 3 4 5 6 7 8 9 10 11 12 13 14 15 16 17 18 19 20 21 22 23 24 25 26 27 28 29 30 31

SOMETHING GOOD THAT HAPPENED TODAY
_____
_____
_____
_____

SOMEONE OR SOMETHING I AM THANKFUL FOR AND WHY
_____
_____
_____
_____

MY GOOD DEED, HAPPY THOUGHT, OR KIND ACT FOR THE DAY
_____
_____
_____
_____

> **Be thankful for what you have; you'll end up having more. If you concentrate on what you don't have, you will never, ever have enough.**
> **- Oprah Winfrey**

blessed af

JAN FEB MAR APR MAY JUN JUL AUG SEP OCT NOV DEC
1 2 3 4 5 6 7 8 9 10 11 12 13 14 15 16 17 18 19 20 21 22 23 24 25 26 27 28 29 30 31

SOMETHING GOOD THAT HAPPENED TODAY

_____
_____
_____
_____

SOMEONE OR SOMETHING I AM THANKFUL FOR AND WHY

_____
_____
_____
_____

MY GOOD DEED, HAPPY THOUGHT, OR KIND ACT FOR THE DAY

_____
_____
_____
_____

Above all, be the heroine of your life, not the victim.
- Nora Ephron

blessed af

JAN FEB MAR APR MAY JUN JUL AUG SEP OCT NOV DEC
1 2 3 4 5 6 7 8 9 10 11 12 13 14 15 16 17 18 19 20 21 22 23 24 25 26 27 28 29 30 31

SOMETHING GOOD THAT HAPPENED TODAY
_____
_____
_____
_____

SOMEONE OR SOMETHING I AM THANKFUL FOR AND WHY
_____
_____
_____
_____

MY GOOD DEED, HAPPY THOUGHT, OR KIND ACT FOR THE DAY
_____
_____
_____
_____

**When you are grateful, fear disappears and abundance appears.
- Tony Robbins**

blessed af

JAN FEB MAR APR MAY JUN JUL AUG SEP OCT NOV DEC
1 2 3 4 5 6 7 8 9 10 11 12 13 14 15 16 17 18 19 20 21 22 23 24 25 26 27 28 29 30 31

SOMETHING GOOD THAT HAPPENED TODAY

_____
_____
_____
_____

SOMEONE OR SOMETHING I AM THANKFUL FOR AND WHY

_____
_____
_____
_____

MY GOOD DEED, HAPPY THOUGHT, OR KIND ACT FOR THE DAY

_____
_____
_____
_____

Owning our story can be hard but not nearly as difficult as spending our lives running from it.
- Brene Brown

blessed af

JAN FEB MAR APR MAY JUN JUL AUG SEP OCT NOV DEC
1 2 3 4 5 6 7 8 9 10 11 12 13 14 15 16 17 18 19 20 21 22 23 24 25 26 27 28 29 30 31

SOMETHING GOOD THAT HAPPENED TODAY
_____
_____
_____
_____

SOMEONE OR SOMETHING I AM THANKFUL FOR AND WHY
_____
_____
_____
_____

MY GOOD DEED, HAPPY THOUGHT, OR KIND ACT FOR THE DAY
_____
_____
_____
_____

> Beauty comes from a life well lived. If you've lived well, your smile lines are in the right places, and your frown lines aren't too bad, what more do you need?
> - Jennifer Garner

blessed af

JAN FEB MAR APR MAY JUN JUL AUG SEP OCT NOV DEC
1 2 3 4 5 6 7 8 9 10 11 12 13 14 15 16 17 18 19 20 21 22 23 24 25 26 27 28 29 30 31

SOMETHING GOOD THAT HAPPENED TODAY
_____
_____
_____
_____

SOMEONE OR SOMETHING I AM THANKFUL FOR AND WHY
_____
_____
_____
_____

MY GOOD DEED, HAPPY THOUGHT, OR KIND ACT FOR THE DAY
_____
_____
_____
_____

Feeling gratitude and not expressing it is like wrapping a present and not giving it.
- William Arthur Ward

blessed af

JAN FEB MAR APR MAY JUN JUL AUG SEP OCT NOV DEC
1 2 3 4 5 6 7 8 9 10 11 12 13 14 15 16 17 18 19 20 21 22 23 24 25 26 27 28 29 30 31

SOMETHING GOOD THAT HAPPENED TODAY
_____
_____
_____
_____

SOMEONE OR SOMETHING I AM THANKFUL FOR AND WHY
_____
_____
_____
_____

MY GOOD DEED, HAPPY THOUGHT, OR KIND ACT FOR THE DAY
_____
_____
_____
_____

You can't be that kid standing at the top of the waterslide, overthinking it. You have to go down the chute.
- Tina Fey

blessed af

JAN FEB MAR APR MAY JUN JUL AUG SEP OCT NOV DEC
1 2 3 4 5 6 7 8 9 10 11 12 13 14 15 16 17 18 19 20 21 22 23 24 25 26 27 28 29 30 31

SOMETHING GOOD THAT HAPPENED TODAY

_____
_____
_____
_____

SOMEONE OR SOMETHING I AM THANKFUL FOR AND WHY

_____
_____
_____
_____

MY GOOD DEED, HAPPY THOUGHT, OR KIND ACT FOR THE DAY

_____
_____
_____
_____

Gratitude is an antidote to negative emotions, a neutralizer of envy, hostility, worry, and irritation. It is savoring; it is not taking things for granted; it is present-oriented.
- Sonja Lyubomirsky

blessed af

JAN FEB MAR APR MAY JUN JUL AUG SEP OCT NOV DEC
1 2 3 4 5 6 7 8 9 10 11 12 13 14 15 16 17 18 19 20 21 22 23 24 25 26 27 28 29 30 31

SOMETHING GOOD THAT HAPPENED TODAY
_____
_____
_____
_____

SOMEONE OR SOMETHING I AM THANKFUL FOR AND WHY
_____
_____
_____
_____

MY GOOD DEED, HAPPY THOUGHT, OR KIND ACT FOR THE DAY
_____
_____
_____
_____

> There are two kinds of people, those who do the work and those who take the credit. Try to be in the first group; there is less competition there.
> - Indira Gandhi

blessed af

JAN FEB MAR APR MAY JUN JUL AUG SEP OCT NOV DEC
1 2 3 4 5 6 7 8 9 10 11 12 13 14 15 16 17 18 19 20 21 22 23 24 25 26 27 28 29 30 31

SOMETHING GOOD THAT HAPPENED TODAY

_____
_____
_____
_____

SOMEONE OR SOMETHING I AM THANKFUL FOR AND WHY

_____
_____
_____
_____

MY GOOD DEED, HAPPY THOUGHT, OR KIND ACT FOR THE DAY

_____
_____
_____
_____

The more grateful I am, the more beauty I see.
- Mary Davis

… # blessed af

JAN FEB MAR APR MAY JUN JUL AUG SEP OCT NOV DEC
1 2 3 4 5 6 7 8 9 10 11 12 13 14 15 16 17 18 19 20 21 22 23 24 25 26 27 28 29 30 31

SOMETHING GOOD THAT HAPPENED TODAY
_____
_____
_____
_____

SOMEONE OR SOMETHING I AM THANKFUL
FOR AND WHY
_____
_____
_____
_____

MY GOOD DEED, HAPPY THOUGHT, OR
KIND ACT FOR THE DAY
_____
_____
_____
_____

**When you're through changing,
you're through.
- Martha Stewart**

blessed af

JAN FEB MAR APR MAY JUN JUL AUG SEP OCT NOV DEC
1 2 3 4 5 6 7 8 9 10 11 12 13 14 15 16 17 18 19 20 21 22 23 24 25 26 27 28 29 30 31

SOMETHING GOOD THAT HAPPENED TODAY

_____
_____
_____
_____

SOMEONE OR SOMETHING I AM THANKFUL FOR AND WHY

_____
_____
_____
_____

MY GOOD DEED, HAPPY THOUGHT, OR KIND ACT FOR THE DAY

_____
_____
_____
_____

Gratitude is the healthiest of all human emotions. The more you express gratitude for what you have, the more likely you will have even more to express gratitude for.
- Zig Ziglar

blessed af

JAN FEB MAR APR MAY JUN JUL AUG SEP OCT NOV DEC
1 2 3 4 5 6 7 8 9 10 11 12 13 14 15 16 17 18 19 20 21 22 23 24 25 26 27 28 29 30 31

SOMETHING GOOD THAT HAPPENED TODAY
_____
_____
_____
_____

SOMEONE OR SOMETHING I AM THANKFUL FOR AND WHY
_____
_____
_____
_____

MY GOOD DEED, HAPPY THOUGHT, OR KIND ACT FOR THE DAY
_____
_____
_____
_____

Whenever you are blue or lonely or stricken by some humiliating thing you did, the cure and the hope is in caring about other people.
- Diane Sawyer

blessed af

JAN FEB MAR APR MAY JUN JUL AUG SEP OCT NOV DEC
1 2 3 4 5 6 7 8 9 10 11 12 13 14 15 16 17 18 19 20 21 22 23 24 25 26 27 28 29 30 31

SOMETHING GOOD THAT HAPPENED TODAY

_____
_____
_____
_____

SOMEONE OR SOMETHING I AM THANKFUL FOR AND WHY

_____
_____
_____
_____

MY GOOD DEED, HAPPY THOUGHT, OR KIND ACT FOR THE DAY

_____
_____
_____
_____

> **When I'm tired, I rest. I say, 'I can't be a superwoman today.'**
> **- Jada Pinkett Smith**

blessed af

JAN FEB MAR APR MAY JUN JUL AUG SEP OCT NOV DEC
1 2 3 4 5 6 7 8 9 10 11 12 13 14 15 16 17 18 19 20 21 22 23 24 25 26 27 28 29 30 31

SOMETHING GOOD THAT HAPPENED TODAY
_____
_____
_____
_____

SOMEONE OR SOMETHING I AM THANKFUL FOR AND WHY
_____
_____
_____
_____

MY GOOD DEED, HAPPY THOUGHT, OR KIND ACT FOR THE DAY
_____
_____
_____
_____

> Gratitude makes sense of our past, brings peace for today, and creates a vision for tomorrow.
> - Melody Beattie

blessed af

JAN FEB MAR APR MAY JUN JUL AUG SEP OCT NOV DEC
1 2 3 4 5 6 7 8 9 10 11 12 13 14 15 16 17 18 19 20 21 22 23 24 25 26 27 28 29 30 31

SOMETHING GOOD THAT HAPPENED TODAY
_____
_____
_____
_____

SOMEONE OR SOMETHING I AM THANKFUL FOR AND WHY
_____
_____
_____
_____

MY GOOD DEED, HAPPY THOUGHT, OR KIND ACT FOR THE DAY
_____
_____
_____
_____

Do what you feel in your heart to be right—for you'll be criticized anyway.
- Eleanor Roosevelt

blessed af

JAN FEB MAR APR MAY JUN JUL AUG SEP OCT NOV DEC
1 2 3 4 5 6 7 8 9 10 11 12 13 14 15 16 17 18 19 20 21 22 23 24 25 26 27 28 29 30 31

SOMETHING GOOD THAT HAPPENED TODAY
_____
_____
_____
_____

SOMEONE OR SOMETHING I AM THANKFUL FOR AND WHY
_____
_____
_____
_____

MY GOOD DEED, HAPPY THOUGHT, OR KIND ACT FOR THE DAY
_____
_____
_____
_____

Sometimes life knocks you on your ass... get up, get up, get up!!! Happiness is not the absence of problems, it's the ability to deal with them.
- Steve Maraboli

blessed af

JAN FEB MAR APR MAY JUN JUL AUG SEP OCT NOV DEC
1 2 3 4 5 6 7 8 9 10 11 12 13 14 15 16 17 18 19 20 21 22 23 24 25 26 27 28 29 30 31

SOMETHING GOOD THAT HAPPENED TODAY
_____
_____
_____
_____

SOMEONE OR SOMETHING I AM THANKFUL FOR AND WHY
_____
_____
_____
_____

MY GOOD DEED, HAPPY THOUGHT, OR KIND ACT FOR THE DAY
_____
_____
_____
_____

Thankfulness may consist merely of words. Gratitude is shown in acts.
- Henri Frederic Amiel

blessed af

JAN FEB MAR APR MAY JUN JUL AUG SEP OCT NOV DEC
1 2 3 4 5 6 7 8 9 10 11 12 13 14 15 16 17 18 19 20 21 22 23 24 25 26 27 28 29 30 31

SOMETHING GOOD THAT HAPPENED TODAY
_____
_____
_____
_____

SOMEONE OR SOMETHING I AM THANKFUL FOR AND WHY
_____
_____
_____
_____

MY GOOD DEED, HAPPY THOUGHT, OR KIND ACT FOR THE DAY
_____
_____
_____
_____

> In ordinary life, we hardly realize that we receive a great deal more than we give, and that it is only with gratitude that life becomes rich.
> - Dietrich Bonhoeffer

blessed af

JAN FEB MAR APR MAY JUN JUL AUG SEP OCT NOV DEC
1 2 3 4 5 6 7 8 9 10 11 12 13 14 15 16 17 18 19 20 21 22 23 24 25 26 27 28 29 30 31

SOMETHING GOOD THAT HAPPENED TODAY

___

SOMEONE OR SOMETHING I AM THANKFUL FOR AND WHY

___

MY GOOD DEED, HAPPY THOUGHT, OR KIND ACT FOR THE DAY

___

Character cannot be developed in ease and quiet. Only through experience of trial and suffering can the soul be strengthened, ambition inspired, and success achieved.
- Helen Keller

blessed af

JAN FEB MAR APR MAY JUN JUL AUG SEP OCT NOV DEC
1 2 3 4 5 6 7 8 9 10 11 12 13 14 15 16 17 18 19 20 21 22 23 24 25 26 27 28 29 30 31

SOMETHING GOOD THAT HAPPENED TODAY
_____
_____
_____
_____

SOMEONE OR SOMETHING I AM THANKFUL FOR AND WHY
_____
_____
_____
_____

MY GOOD DEED, HAPPY THOUGHT, OR KIND ACT FOR THE DAY
_____
_____
_____
_____

> If you think taking care of yourself is selfish, change your mind. If you don't, you're simply ducking your responsibilities.
> - Ann Richards

blessed af

JAN FEB MAR APR MAY JUN JUL AUG SEP OCT NOV DEC
1 2 3 4 5 6 7 8 9 10 11 12 13 14 15 16 17 18 19 20 21 22 23 24 25 26 27 28 29 30 31

SOMETHING GOOD THAT HAPPENED TODAY

_____
_____
_____
_____

SOMEONE OR SOMETHING I AM THANKFUL FOR AND WHY

_____
_____
_____
_____

MY GOOD DEED, HAPPY THOUGHT, OR KIND ACT FOR THE DAY

_____
_____
_____
_____

The deepest craving of human nature is the need to be appreciated.
- William James

blessed af

JAN FEB MAR APR MAY JUN JUL AUG SEP OCT NOV DEC
1 2 3 4 5 6 7 8 9 10 11 12 13 14 15 16 17 18 19 20 21 22 23 24 25 26 27 28 29 30 31

SOMETHING GOOD THAT HAPPENED TODAY
_____
_____
_____
_____

SOMEONE OR SOMETHING I AM THANKFUL FOR AND WHY
_____
_____
_____
_____

MY GOOD DEED, HAPPY THOUGHT, OR KIND ACT FOR THE DAY
_____
_____
_____
_____

**Gratitude is the most exquisite form of courtesy.
- Jacques Maritain**

blessed af

JAN FEB MAR APR MAY JUN JUL AUG SEP OCT NOV DEC
1 2 3 4 5 6 7 8 9 10 11 12 13 14 15 16 17 18 19 20 21 22 23 24 25 26 27 28 29 30 31

SOMETHING GOOD THAT HAPPENED TODAY

_____
_____
_____
_____

SOMEONE OR SOMETHING I AM THANKFUL FOR AND WHY

_____
_____
_____
_____

MY GOOD DEED, HAPPY THOUGHT, OR KIND ACT FOR THE DAY

_____
_____
_____
_____

Well-behaved women seldom make history.
- Laurel Thatcher Ulrich

blessed af

JAN FEB MAR APR MAY JUN JUL AUG SEP OCT NOV DEC
1 2 3 4 5 6 7 8 9 10 11 12 13 14 15 16 17 18 19 20 21 22 23 24 25 26 27 28 29 30 31

SOMETHING GOOD THAT HAPPENED TODAY
_____
_____
_____
_____

SOMEONE OR SOMETHING I AM THANKFUL FOR AND WHY
_____
_____
_____
_____

MY GOOD DEED, HAPPY THOUGHT, OR KIND ACT FOR THE DAY
_____
_____
_____
_____

> Gratitude unlocks the fullness of life. It turns what we have into enough, and more. It turns denial into acceptance, chaos to order, confusion to clarity. It can turn a meal into a feast, a house into a home, a stranger into a friend.
> - Melody Beattie

blessed af

JAN FEB MAR APR MAY JUN JUL AUG SEP OCT NOV DEC
1 2 3 4 5 6 7 8 9 10 11 12 13 14 15 16 17 18 19 20 21 22 23 24 25 26 27 28 29 30 31

SOMETHING GOOD THAT HAPPENED TODAY

_____
_____
_____
_____

SOMEONE OR SOMETHING I AM THANKFUL FOR AND WHY

_____
_____
_____
_____

MY GOOD DEED, HAPPY THOUGHT, OR KIND ACT FOR THE DAY

_____
_____
_____
_____

We can only be said to be alive in those moments when our hearts are conscious of our treasures.
- Thornton Wilder

blessed af

JAN FEB MAR APR MAY JUN JUL AUG SEP OCT NOV DEC
1 2 3 4 5 6 7 8 9 10 11 12 13 14 15 16 17 18 19 20 21 22 23 24 25 26 27 28 29 30 31

SOMETHING GOOD THAT HAPPENED TODAY
_____
_____
_____
_____

SOMEONE OR SOMETHING I AM THANKFUL FOR AND WHY
_____
_____
_____
_____

MY GOOD DEED, HAPPY THOUGHT, OR KIND ACT FOR THE DAY
_____
_____
_____
_____

**When you feel your best, everybody else can feel it too.
- Ariana Grande**

blessed af

JAN FEB MAR APR MAY JUN JUL AUG SEP OCT NOV DEC
1 2 3 4 5 6 7 8 9 10 11 12 13 14 15 16 17 18 19 20 21 22 23 24 25 26 27 28 29 30 31

SOMETHING GOOD THAT HAPPENED TODAY
_____
_____
_____
_____

SOMEONE OR SOMETHING I AM THANKFUL FOR AND WHY
_____
_____
_____
_____

MY GOOD DEED, HAPPY THOUGHT, OR KIND ACT FOR THE DAY
_____
_____
_____
_____

**As we express our gratitude, we must never forget that the highest appreciation is not to utter words, but to live by them.
- John F. Kennedy**

blessed af

JAN FEB MAR APR MAY JUN JUL AUG SEP OCT NOV DEC
1 2 3 4 5 6 7 8 9 10 11 12 13 14 15 16 17 18 19 20 21 22 23 24 25 26 27 28 29 30 31

SOMETHING GOOD THAT HAPPENED TODAY
_____
_____
_____
_____

SOMEONE OR SOMETHING I AM THANKFUL FOR AND WHY
_____
_____
_____
_____

MY GOOD DEED, HAPPY THOUGHT, OR KIND ACT FOR THE DAY
_____
_____
_____
_____

Gratitude is riches.
Complaint is poverty.
- Doris Day

blessed af

JAN FEB MAR APR MAY JUN JUL AUG SEP OCT NOV DEC
1 2 3 4 5 6 7 8 9 10 11 12 13 14 15 16 17 18 19 20 21 22 23 24 25 26 27 28 29 30 31

SOMETHING GOOD THAT HAPPENED TODAY

_____
_____
_____
_____

SOMEONE OR SOMETHING I AM THANKFUL FOR AND WHY

_____
_____
_____
_____

MY GOOD DEED, HAPPY THOUGHT, OR KIND ACT FOR THE DAY

_____
_____
_____
_____

> 'Thank you' is the best prayer that anyone could say. I say that one a lot. Thank you expresses extreme gratitude, humility, understanding.
> - Alice Walker

blessed af

JAN FEB MAR APR MAY JUN JUL AUG SEP OCT NOV DEC
1 2 3 4 5 6 7 8 9 10 11 12 13 14 15 16 17 18 19 20 21 22 23 24 25 26 27 28 29 30 31

SOMETHING GOOD THAT HAPPENED TODAY
_____
_____
_____
_____
_____

SOMEONE OR SOMETHING I AM THANKFUL FOR AND WHY
_____
_____
_____
_____
_____

MY GOOD DEED, HAPPY THOUGHT, OR KIND ACT FOR THE DAY
_____
_____
_____
_____
_____

> Entitlement is a happiness killer.
> When we aren't giving thanks for things, we're feeling entitled to them.
> - Greg Boyd

blessed af

JAN FEB MAR APR MAY JUN JUL AUG SEP OCT NOV DEC
1 2 3 4 5 6 7 8 9 10 11 12 13 14 15 16 17 18 19 20 21 22 23 24 25 26 27 28 29 30 31

SOMETHING GOOD THAT HAPPENED TODAY

SOMEONE OR SOMETHING I AM THANKFUL FOR AND WHY

MY GOOD DEED, HAPPY THOUGHT, OR KIND ACT FOR THE DAY

It's the messy parts that make us human, so we should embrace them too — pat ourselves on the back for getting through them rather than being angry for having gotten into them in the first place.
- Jennifer Lopez

blessed af

JAN FEB MAR APR MAY JUN JUL AUG SEP OCT NOV DEC
1 2 3 4 5 6 7 8 9 10 11 12 13 14 15 16 17 18 19 20 21 22 23 24 25 26 27 28 29 30 31

SOMETHING GOOD THAT HAPPENED TODAY
_____
_____
_____
_____

SOMEONE OR SOMETHING I AM THANKFUL FOR AND WHY
_____
_____
_____
_____

MY GOOD DEED, HAPPY THOUGHT, OR KIND ACT FOR THE DAY
_____
_____
_____
_____

> There are only two ways to live your life. One is as though nothing is a miracle. The other is as though everything is a miracle.
> - Albert Einstein

blessed af

JAN FEB MAR APR MAY JUN JUL AUG SEP OCT NOV DEC
1 2 3 4 5 6 7 8 9 10 11 12 13 14 15 16 17 18 19 20 21 22 23 24 25 26 27 28 29 30 31

SOMETHING GOOD THAT HAPPENED TODAY

_____
_____
_____
_____

SOMEONE OR SOMETHING I AM THANKFUL FOR AND WHY

_____
_____
_____
_____

MY GOOD DEED, HAPPY THOUGHT, OR KIND ACT FOR THE DAY

_____
_____
_____
_____

It's not having what you want, it's wanting what you've got.
- Sheryl Crow

blessed af

JAN FEB MAR APR MAY JUN JUL AUG SEP OCT NOV DEC
1 2 3 4 5 6 7 8 9 10 11 12 13 14 15 16 17 18 19 20 21 22 23 24 25 26 27 28 29 30 31

SOMETHING GOOD THAT HAPPENED TODAY
___
___
___
___

SOMEONE OR SOMETHING I AM THANKFUL FOR AND WHY
___
___
___
___

MY GOOD DEED, HAPPY THOUGHT, OR KIND ACT FOR THE DAY
___
___
___
___

Some people grumble that roses have thorns; I am grateful that thorns have roses.
- Alphonse Karr

blessed af

JAN FEB MAR APR MAY JUN JUL AUG SEP OCT NOV DEC
1 2 3 4 5 6 7 8 9 10 11 12 13 14 15 16 17 18 19 20 21 22 23 24 25 26 27 28 29 30 31

SOMETHING GOOD THAT HAPPENED TODAY

_____
_____
_____
_____

SOMEONE OR SOMETHING I AM THANKFUL FOR AND WHY

_____
_____
_____
_____

MY GOOD DEED, HAPPY THOUGHT, OR KIND ACT FOR THE DAY

_____
_____
_____
_____

The way we respond to things is a big indicator of our character and what type of person we are.
- Zendaya

blessed af

| JAN | FEB | MAR | APR | MAY | JUN | JUL | AUG | SEP | OCT | NOV | DEC |

1 2 3 4 5 6 7 8 9 10 11 12 13 14 15 16 17 18 19 20 21 22 23 24 25 26 27 28 29 30 31

SOMETHING GOOD THAT HAPPENED TODAY

_____
_____
_____
_____

SOMEONE OR SOMETHING I AM THANKFUL FOR AND WHY

_____
_____
_____
_____

MY GOOD DEED, HAPPY THOUGHT, OR KIND ACT FOR THE DAY

_____
_____
_____
_____

> It's a funny thing about life, once you begin to take note of the things you are grateful for, you begin to lose sight of the things that you lack.
> - Germany Kent

blessed af

JAN FEB MAR APR MAY JUN JUL AUG SEP OCT NOV DEC
1 2 3 4 5 6 7 8 9 10 11 12 13 14 15 16 17 18 19 20 21 22 23 24 25 26 27 28 29 30 31

SOMETHING GOOD THAT HAPPENED TODAY

_____
_____
_____
_____

SOMEONE OR SOMETHING I AM THANKFUL FOR AND WHY

_____
_____
_____
_____

MY GOOD DEED, HAPPY THOUGHT, OR KIND ACT FOR THE DAY

_____
_____
_____
_____

The heart that gives thanks is a happy one, for we cannot feel thankful and unhappy at the same time.
- Douglas Wood

blessed af

| JAN | FEB | MAR | APR | MAY | JUN | JUL | AUG | SEP | OCT | NOV | DEC |

1 2 3 4 5 6 7 8 9 10 11 12 13 14 15 16 17 18 19 20 21 22 23 24 25 26 27 28 29 30 31

SOMETHING GOOD THAT HAPPENED TODAY

_____
_____
_____
_____

SOMEONE OR SOMETHING I AM THANKFUL FOR AND WHY

_____
_____
_____
_____

MY GOOD DEED, HAPPY THOUGHT, OR KIND ACT FOR THE DAY

_____
_____
_____
_____

> Follow your passion. Stay true to yourself. Never follow someone else's path unless you're in the woods and you're lost and you see a path. By all means, you should follow that.
> - Ellen DeGeneres

blessed af

JAN FEB MAR APR MAY JUN JUL AUG SEP OCT NOV DEC
1 2 3 4 5 6 7 8 9 10 11 12 13 14 15 16 17 18 19 20 21 22 23 24 25 26 27 28 29 30 31

SOMETHING GOOD THAT HAPPENED TODAY

_____
_____
_____
_____

SOMEONE OR SOMETHING I AM THANKFUL FOR AND WHY

_____
_____
_____
_____

MY GOOD DEED, HAPPY THOUGHT, OR KIND ACT FOR THE DAY

_____
_____
_____
_____

Piglet noticed that even though he had a very small Heart, it could hold a rather large amount of Gratitude.
- A.A. Milne

blessed af

JAN FEB MAR APR MAY JUN JUL AUG SEP OCT NOV DEC
1 2 3 4 5 6 7 8 9 10 11 12 13 14 15 16 17 18 19 20 21 22 23 24 25 26 27 28 29 30 31

SOMETHING GOOD THAT HAPPENED TODAY
_____
_____
_____
_____

SOMEONE OR SOMETHING I AM THANKFUL FOR AND WHY
_____
_____
_____
_____

MY GOOD DEED, HAPPY THOUGHT, OR KIND ACT FOR THE DAY
_____
_____
_____
_____

> Failure is nothing more than life's way of nudging you that you are off course.
> - Sara Blakely

blessed af

JAN FEB MAR APR MAY JUN JUL AUG SEP OCT NOV DEC
1 2 3 4 5 6 7 8 9 10 11 12 13 14 15 16 17 18 19 20 21 22 23 24 25 26 27 28 29 30 31

SOMETHING GOOD THAT HAPPENED TODAY

_____
_____
_____
_____

SOMEONE OR SOMETHING I AM THANKFUL FOR AND WHY

_____
_____
_____
_____

MY GOOD DEED, HAPPY THOUGHT, OR KIND ACT FOR THE DAY

_____
_____
_____
_____

**I love those who can smile in trouble.
- Leonardo da Vinci**

blessed af

JAN FEB MAR APR MAY JUN JUL AUG SEP OCT NOV DEC
1 2 3 4 5 6 7 8 9 10 11 12 13 14 15 16 17 18 19 20 21 22 23 24 25 26 27 28 29 30 31

SOMETHING GOOD THAT HAPPENED TODAY
_____
_____
_____
_____

SOMEONE OR SOMETHING I AM THANKFUL FOR AND WHY
_____
_____
_____
_____

MY GOOD DEED, HAPPY THOUGHT, OR KIND ACT FOR THE DAY
_____
_____
_____
_____

True forgiveness is when you can say, 'Thank you for the experience.'
- Oprah

blessed af

JAN FEB MAR APR MAY JUN JUL AUG SEP OCT NOV DEC
1 2 3 4 5 6 7 8 9 10 11 12 13 14 15 16 17 18 19 20 21 22 23 24 25 26 27 28 29 30 31

SOMETHING GOOD THAT HAPPENED TODAY

_____
_____
_____
_____

SOMEONE OR SOMETHING I AM THANKFUL FOR AND WHY

_____
_____
_____
_____

MY GOOD DEED, HAPPY THOUGHT, OR KIND ACT FOR THE DAY

_____
_____
_____
_____

**It is failure that gives you the proper perspective on success.
- Ellen DeGeneres**

blessed af

JAN FEB MAR APR MAY JUN JUL AUG SEP OCT NOV DEC
1 2 3 4 5 6 7 8 9 10 11 12 13 14 15 16 17 18 19 20 21 22 23 24 25 26 27 28 29 30 31

SOMETHING GOOD THAT HAPPENED TODAY
_____
_____
_____
_____

SOMEONE OR SOMETHING I AM THANKFUL FOR AND WHY
_____
_____
_____
_____

MY GOOD DEED, HAPPY THOUGHT, OR KIND ACT FOR THE DAY
_____
_____
_____
_____

The more you are in a state of gratitude, the more you will attract things to be grateful for.
- Walt Disney

blessed af

JAN FEB MAR APR MAY JUN JUL AUG SEP OCT NOV DEC
1 2 3 4 5 6 7 8 9 10 11 12 13 14 15 16 17 18 19 20 21 22 23 24 25 26 27 28 29 30 31

SOMETHING GOOD THAT HAPPENED TODAY

_____
_____
_____
_____

SOMEONE OR SOMETHING I AM THANKFUL FOR AND WHY

_____
_____
_____
_____

MY GOOD DEED, HAPPY THOUGHT, OR KIND ACT FOR THE DAY

_____
_____
_____
_____

Don't be fooled by this game of perfections humans play.
- Kristen Bell

blessed af

JAN FEB MAR APR MAY JUN JUL AUG SEP OCT NOV DEC
1 2 3 4 5 6 7 8 9 10 11 12 13 14 15 16 17 18 19 20 21 22 23 24 25 26 27 28 29 30 31

SOMETHING GOOD THAT HAPPENED TODAY
_____
_____
_____
_____

SOMEONE OR SOMETHING I AM THANKFUL FOR AND WHY
_____
_____
_____
_____

MY GOOD DEED, HAPPY THOUGHT, OR KIND ACT FOR THE DAY
_____
_____
_____
_____

> The unthankful heart discovers no mercies; but the thankful heart will find, in every hour, some heavenly blessings.
> - Henry Ward Beecher

blessed af

JAN FEB MAR APR MAY JUN JUL AUG SEP OCT NOV DEC
1 2 3 4 5 6 7 8 9 10 11 12 13 14 15 16 17 18 19 20 21 22 23 24 25 26 27 28 29 30 31

SOMETHING GOOD THAT HAPPENED TODAY
___
___
___
___

SOMEONE OR SOMETHING I AM THANKFUL FOR AND WHY
___
___
___
___

MY GOOD DEED, HAPPY THOUGHT, OR KIND ACT FOR THE DAY
___
___
___
___

**Be happy being you.
- Ariana Grande**

blessed af

| JAN | FEB | MAR | APR | MAY | JUN | JUL | AUG | SEP | OCT | NOV | DEC |

1 2 3 4 5 6 7 8 9 10 11 12 13 14 15 16 17 18 19 20 21 22 23 24 25 26 27 28 29 30 31

SOMETHING GOOD THAT HAPPENED TODAY
_____
_____
_____
_____

SOMEONE OR SOMETHING I AM THANKFUL FOR AND WHY
_____
_____
_____
_____

MY GOOD DEED, HAPPY THOUGHT, OR KIND ACT FOR THE DAY
_____
_____
_____
_____

> **Only you can decide what you become.**
> **- Seth Adam Smith**

blessed af

JAN FEB MAR APR MAY JUN JUL AUG SEP OCT NOV DEC
1 2 3 4 5 6 7 8 9 10 11 12 13 14 15 16 17 18 19 20 21 22 23 24 25 26 27 28 29 30 31

SOMETHING GOOD THAT HAPPENED TODAY
_____
_____
_____
_____

SOMEONE OR SOMETHING I AM THANKFUL FOR AND WHY
_____
_____
_____
_____

MY GOOD DEED, HAPPY THOUGHT, OR KIND ACT FOR THE DAY
_____
_____
_____
_____

Get at least eight hours of beauty sleep, nine if you're ugly.
- Betty White

blessed af

JAN FEB MAR APR MAY JUN JUL AUG SEP OCT NOV DEC
1 2 3 4 5 6 7 8 9 10 11 12 13 14 15 16 17 18 19 20 21 22 23 24 25 26 27 28 29 30 31

SOMETHING GOOD THAT HAPPENED TODAY
_____
_____
_____
_____

SOMEONE OR SOMETHING I AM THANKFUL
FOR AND WHY
_____
_____
_____
_____

MY GOOD DEED, HAPPY THOUGHT, OR
KIND ACT FOR THE DAY
_____
_____
_____
_____

> Gratitude is the ability to experience life as a gift. It liberates us from the prison of self-preoccupation.
> - John Ortberg

blessed af

JAN FEB MAR APR MAY JUN JUL AUG SEP OCT NOV DEC
1 2 3 4 5 6 7 8 9 10 11 12 13 14 15 16 17 18 19 20 21 22 23 24 25 26 27 28 29 30 31

SOMETHING GOOD THAT HAPPENED TODAY
_____
_____
_____
_____

SOMEONE OR SOMETHING I AM THANKFUL FOR AND WHY
_____
_____
_____
_____

MY GOOD DEED, HAPPY THOUGHT, OR KIND ACT FOR THE DAY
_____
_____
_____
_____

> The soul that gives thanks can find comfort in everything; the soul that complains can find comfort in nothing.
> - Hannah Whitall Smith

blessed af

JAN FEB MAR APR MAY JUN JUL AUG SEP OCT NOV DEC
1 2 3 4 5 6 7 8 9 10 11 12 13 14 15 16 17 18 19 20 21 22 23 24 25 26 27 28 29 30 31

SOMETHING GOOD THAT HAPPENED TODAY

_____
_____
_____
_____

SOMEONE OR SOMETHING I AM THANKFUL FOR AND WHY

_____
_____
_____
_____

MY GOOD DEED, HAPPY THOUGHT, OR KIND ACT FOR THE DAY

_____
_____
_____
_____

> There are two primary choices in life; to accept conditions as they exist, or accept the responsibility for changing them.
> - Denis Waitley

blessed af

JAN FEB MAR APR MAY JUN JUL AUG SEP OCT NOV DEC
1 2 3 4 5 6 7 8 9 10 11 12 13 14 15 16 17 18 19 20 21 22 23 24 25 26 27 28 29 30 31

SOMETHING GOOD THAT HAPPENED TODAY
_____
_____
_____
_____

SOMEONE OR SOMETHING I AM THANKFUL FOR AND WHY
_____
_____
_____
_____

MY GOOD DEED, HAPPY THOUGHT, OR KIND ACT FOR THE DAY
_____
_____
_____
_____

Things don't always turn out exactly the way you want them to be and you feel disappointed. You are not always going to be the winner. That's when you have to stop and figure out why things happened the way they did and what you can do to change them.
- Jennifer Lopez

blessed af

| JAN | FEB | MAR | APR | MAY | JUN | JUL | AUG | SEP | OCT | NOV | DEC |

1 2 3 4 5 6 7 8 9 10 11 12 13 14 15 16 17 18 19 20 21 22 23 24 25 26 27 28 29 30 31

SOMETHING GOOD THAT HAPPENED TODAY
___
___
___
___

SOMEONE OR SOMETHING I AM THANKFUL FOR AND WHY
___
___
___
___

MY GOOD DEED, HAPPY THOUGHT, OR KIND ACT FOR THE DAY
___
___
___
___

Gratitude and attitude are not challenges; they are choices.
- Robert Braathe

blessed af

JAN FEB MAR APR MAY JUN JUL AUG SEP OCT NOV DEC
1 2 3 4 5 6 7 8 9 10 11 12 13 14 15 16 17 18 19 20 21 22 23 24 25 26 27 28 29 30 31

SOMETHING GOOD THAT HAPPENED TODAY

_____
_____
_____
_____

SOMEONE OR SOMETHING I AM THANKFUL FOR AND WHY

_____
_____
_____
_____

MY GOOD DEED, HAPPY THOUGHT, OR KIND ACT FOR THE DAY

_____
_____
_____
_____

> We can only be said to be alive in those moments when our hearts are conscious of our treasures.
> - Thornton Wilder

blessed af

JAN FEB MAR APR MAY JUN JUL AUG SEP OCT NOV DEC
1 2 3 4 5 6 7 8 9 10 11 12 13 14 15 16 17 18 19 20 21 22 23 24 25 26 27 28 29 30 31

SOMETHING GOOD THAT HAPPENED TODAY
_____
_____
_____
_____

SOMEONE OR SOMETHING I AM THANKFUL FOR AND WHY
_____
_____
_____
_____

MY GOOD DEED, HAPPY THOUGHT, OR KIND ACT FOR THE DAY
_____
_____
_____
_____

Rock bottom became the solid foundation on which I rebuilt my life.
- J.K. Rowling

blessed af

JAN FEB MAR APR MAY JUN JUL AUG SEP OCT NOV DEC
1 2 3 4 5 6 7 8 9 10 11 12 13 14 15 16 17 18 19 20 21 22 23 24 25 26 27 28 29 30 31

SOMETHING GOOD THAT HAPPENED TODAY

_____
_____
_____
_____

SOMEONE OR SOMETHING I AM THANKFUL FOR AND WHY

_____
_____
_____
_____

MY GOOD DEED, HAPPY THOUGHT, OR KIND ACT FOR THE DAY

_____
_____
_____
_____

> **Gratitude goes beyond the 'mine' and 'thine' and claims the truth that all of life is a pure gift.**
> **- Henri J.M. Nouwen**

blessed af

| JAN | FEB | MAR | APR | MAY | JUN | JUL | AUG | SEP | OCT | NOV | DEC |

1 2 3 4 5 6 7 8 9 10 11 12 13 14 15 16 17 18 19 20 21 22 23 24 25 26 27 28 29 30 31

SOMETHING GOOD THAT HAPPENED TODAY
_____
_____
_____
_____

SOMEONE OR SOMETHING I AM THANKFUL FOR AND WHY
_____
_____
_____
_____

MY GOOD DEED, HAPPY THOUGHT, OR KIND ACT FOR THE DAY
_____
_____
_____
_____

I attribute my success to this: I never gave or took an excuse.
- Florence Nightingale

blessed af

JAN FEB MAR APR MAY JUN JUL AUG SEP OCT NOV DEC
1 2 3 4 5 6 7 8 9 10 11 12 13 14 15 16 17 18 19 20 21 22 23 24 25 26 27 28 29 30 31

SOMETHING GOOD THAT HAPPENED TODAY

_____
_____
_____
_____

SOMEONE OR SOMETHING I AM THANKFUL FOR AND WHY

_____
_____
_____
_____

MY GOOD DEED, HAPPY THOUGHT, OR KIND ACT FOR THE DAY

_____
_____
_____
_____

Don't compromise yourself. You are all you've got.
- Janis Joplin

blessed af

JAN FEB MAR APR MAY JUN JUL AUG SEP OCT NOV DEC
1 2 3 4 5 6 7 8 9 10 11 12 13 14 15 16 17 18 19 20 21 22 23 24 25 26 27 28 29 30 31

SOMETHING GOOD THAT HAPPENED TODAY
_____
_____
_____
_____
_____

SOMEONE OR SOMETHING I AM THANKFUL
FOR AND WHY
_____
_____
_____
_____
_____

MY GOOD DEED, HAPPY THOUGHT, OR
KIND ACT FOR THE DAY
_____
_____
_____
_____
_____

**Sometimes you have to be a bitch to
get things done.
- Madonna**

blessed af

JAN FEB MAR APR MAY JUN JUL AUG SEP OCT NOV DEC
1 2 3 4 5 6 7 8 9 10 11 12 13 14 15 16 17 18 19 20 21 22 23 24 25 26 27 28 29 30 31

SOMETHING GOOD THAT HAPPENED TODAY

_____
_____
_____
_____

SOMEONE OR SOMETHING I AM THANKFUL FOR AND WHY

_____
_____
_____
_____

MY GOOD DEED, HAPPY THOUGHT, OR KIND ACT FOR THE DAY

_____
_____
_____
_____

Success is a great deodorant.
- Elizabeth Taylor

blessed af

JAN FEB MAR APR MAY JUN JUL AUG SEP OCT NOV DEC
1 2 3 4 5 6 7 8 9 10 11 12 13 14 15 16 17 18 19 20 21 22 23 24 25 26 27 28 29 30 31

SOMETHING GOOD THAT HAPPENED TODAY

_____
_____
_____
_____

SOMEONE OR SOMETHING I AM THANKFUL FOR AND WHY

_____
_____
_____
_____

MY GOOD DEED, HAPPY THOUGHT, OR KIND ACT FOR THE DAY

_____
_____
_____
_____

Yesterday is history, tomorrow is a mystery, today is a gift of God, which is why we call it the present.
- Bill Keane

blessed af

JAN FEB MAR APR MAY JUN JUL AUG SEP OCT NOV DEC
1 2 3 4 5 6 7 8 9 10 11 12 13 14 15 16 17 18 19 20 21 22 23 24 25 26 27 28 29 30 31

SOMETHING GOOD THAT HAPPENED TODAY

___

SOMEONE OR SOMETHING I AM THANKFUL FOR AND WHY

___

MY GOOD DEED, HAPPY THOUGHT, OR KIND ACT FOR THE DAY

___

**I have not failed. I've just found 10,000 ways that won't work.
- Thomas A. Edison**

blessed af

JAN　FEB　MAR　APR　MAY　JUN　JUL　AUG　SEP　OCT　NOV　DEC
1　2　3　4　5　6　7　8　9　10　11　12　13　14　15　16　17　18　19　20　21　22　23　24　25　26　27　28　29　30　31

SOMETHING GOOD THAT HAPPENED TODAY
___
___
___
___

SOMEONE OR SOMETHING I AM THANKFUL FOR AND WHY
___
___
___
___

MY GOOD DEED, HAPPY THOUGHT, OR KIND ACT FOR THE DAY
___
___
___
___

> You have brains in your head. You have feet in your shoes. You can steer yourself any direction you choose. You're on your own. And you know what you know. And YOU are the one who'll decide where to go.
> - Dr. Seuss

blessed af

JAN   FEB   MAR   APR   MAY   JUN   JUL   AUG   SEP   OCT   NOV   DEC
1 2 3 4 5 6 7 8 9 10 11 12 13 14 15 16 17 18 19 20 21 22 23 24 25 26 27 28 29 30 31

SOMETHING GOOD THAT HAPPENED TODAY
___
___
___
___

SOMEONE OR SOMETHING I AM THANKFUL FOR AND WHY
___
___
___
___

MY GOOD DEED, HAPPY THOUGHT, OR KIND ACT FOR THE DAY
___
___
___
___

**Everything you can imagine is real.
- Pablo Picasso**

blessed af

JAN FEB MAR APR MAY JUN JUL AUG SEP OCT NOV DEC
1 2 3 4 5 6 7 8 9 10 11 12 13 14 15 16 17 18 19 20 21 22 23 24 25 26 27 28 29 30 31

SOMETHING GOOD THAT HAPPENED TODAY
___
___
___
___

SOMEONE OR SOMETHING I AM THANKFUL FOR AND WHY
___
___
___
___

MY GOOD DEED, HAPPY THOUGHT, OR KIND ACT FOR THE DAY
___
___
___
___

Sometimes things have to go wrong in order to go right.
- Sherrilyn Kenyon

blessed af

JAN FEB MAR APR MAY JUN JUL AUG SEP OCT NOV DEC
1 2 3 4 5 6 7 8 9 10 11 12 13 14 15 16 17 18 19 20 21 22 23 24 25 26 27 28 29 30 31

SOMETHING GOOD THAT HAPPENED TODAY
___
___
___
___

SOMEONE OR SOMETHING I AM THANKFUL FOR AND WHY
___
___
___
___

MY GOOD DEED, HAPPY THOUGHT, OR KIND ACT FOR THE DAY
___
___
___
___

> Lord knows every day is not a success. Every year is not a success. You have to celebrate the good.
> - Reese Witherspoon

blessed af

JAN FEB MAR APR MAY JUN JUL AUG SEP OCT NOV DEC
1 2 3 4 5 6 7 8 9 10 11 12 13 14 15 16 17 18 19 20 21 22 23 24 25 26 27 28 29 30 31

SOMETHING GOOD THAT HAPPENED TODAY
_____
_____
_____
_____

SOMEONE OR SOMETHING I AM THANKFUL FOR AND WHY
_____
_____
_____
_____

MY GOOD DEED, HAPPY THOUGHT, OR KIND ACT FOR THE DAY
_____
_____
_____
_____

Things happen to you. But they don't have to happen to your soul.
- Jennifer Lawrence

blessed af

JAN FEB MAR APR MAY JUN JUL AUG SEP OCT NOV DEC
1 2 3 4 5 6 7 8 9 10 11 12 13 14 15 16 17 18 19 20 21 22 23 24 25 26 27 28 29 30 31

SOMETHING GOOD THAT HAPPENED TODAY

_____
_____
_____
_____

SOMEONE OR SOMETHING I AM THANKFUL FOR AND WHY

_____
_____
_____
_____

MY GOOD DEED, HAPPY THOUGHT, OR KIND ACT FOR THE DAY

_____
_____
_____
_____

Just be yourself, there is no one better.
- Taylor Swift

blessed af

JAN FEB MAR APR MAY JUN JUL AUG SEP OCT NOV DEC
1 2 3 4 5 6 7 8 9 10 11 12 13 14 15 16 17 18 19 20 21 22 23 24 25 26 27 28 29 30 31

SOMETHING GOOD THAT HAPPENED TODAY
_____
_____
_____
_____

SOMEONE OR SOMETHING I AM THANKFUL FOR AND WHY
_____
_____
_____
_____

MY GOOD DEED, HAPPY THOUGHT, OR KIND ACT FOR THE DAY
_____
_____
_____
_____

No matter who tells you no, or that you can't do it...you can do it and dreams do come true.
- Sofie Rovenstine

blessed af

JAN FEB MAR APR MAY JUN JUL AUG SEP OCT NOV DEC
1 2 3 4 5 6 7 8 9 10 11 12 13 14 15 16 17 18 19 20 21 22 23 24 25 26 27 28 29 30 31

SOMETHING GOOD THAT HAPPENED TODAY

_____
_____
_____
_____

SOMEONE OR SOMETHING I AM THANKFUL FOR AND WHY

_____
_____
_____
_____

MY GOOD DEED, HAPPY THOUGHT, OR KIND ACT FOR THE DAY

_____
_____
_____
_____

> **If I don't like something that's going on in my life, I change it. And I don't sit and complain about it for a year.**
> **- Kim Kardashian**

blessed af

JAN FEB MAR APR MAY JUN JUL AUG SEP OCT NOV DEC
1 2 3 4 5 6 7 8 9 10 11 12 13 14 15 16 17 18 19 20 21 22 23 24 25 26 27 28 29 30 31

SOMETHING GOOD THAT HAPPENED TODAY

_____
_____
_____
_____

SOMEONE OR SOMETHING I AM THANKFUL FOR AND WHY

_____
_____
_____
_____

MY GOOD DEED, HAPPY THOUGHT, OR KIND ACT FOR THE DAY

_____
_____
_____
_____

> My dad encouraged us to fail. Growing up, he would ask us what we failed at that week. If we didn't have something, he would be disappointed. It changed my mindset at an early age that failure is not the outcome, failure is not trying. Don't be afraid to fail.
> - Sara Blakely

blessed af

JAN FEB MAR APR MAY JUN JUL AUG SEP OCT NOV DEC
1 2 3 4 5 6 7 8 9 10 11 12 13 14 15 16 17 18 19 20 21 22 23 24 25 26 27 28 29 30 31

SOMETHING GOOD THAT HAPPENED TODAY

_____
_____
_____
_____

SOMEONE OR SOMETHING I AM THANKFUL FOR AND WHY

_____
_____
_____
_____

MY GOOD DEED, HAPPY THOUGHT, OR KIND ACT FOR THE DAY

_____
_____
_____
_____

The way I see it, if you want the rainbow, you gotta put up with the rain.
- Dolly Parton

blessed af

JAN FEB MAR APR MAY JUN JUL AUG SEP OCT NOV DEC
1 2 3 4 5 6 7 8 9 10 11 12 13 14 15 16 17 18 19 20 21 22 23 24 25 26 27 28 29 30 31

SOMETHING GOOD THAT HAPPENED TODAY
_____
_____
_____
_____

SOMEONE OR SOMETHING I AM THANKFUL
FOR AND WHY
_____
_____
_____
_____

MY GOOD DEED, HAPPY THOUGHT, OR
KIND ACT FOR THE DAY
_____
_____
_____
_____

**Be thankful for everything that
happens in your life; it's
all experience.
- Roy T. Bennett**

blessed af

JAN FEB MAR APR MAY JUN JUL AUG SEP OCT NOV DEC
1 2 3 4 5 6 7 8 9 10 11 12 13 14 15 16 17 18 19 20 21 22 23 24 25 26 27 28 29 30 31

SOMETHING GOOD THAT HAPPENED TODAY

_____
_____
_____
_____

SOMEONE OR SOMETHING I AM THANKFUL FOR AND WHY

_____
_____
_____
_____

MY GOOD DEED, HAPPY THOUGHT, OR KIND ACT FOR THE DAY

_____
_____
_____
_____

If the only prayer you said was thank you, that would be enough.
- Meister Eckhart

blessed af

JAN   FEB   MAR   APR   MAY   JUN   JUL   AUG   SEP   OCT   NOV   DEC
1 2 3 4 5 6 7 8 9 10 11 12 13 14 15 16 17 18 19 20 21 22 23 24 25 26 27 28 29 30 31

SOMETHING GOOD THAT HAPPENED TODAY
_____
_____
_____
_____

SOMEONE OR SOMETHING I AM THANKFUL FOR AND WHY
_____
_____
_____
_____

MY GOOD DEED, HAPPY THOUGHT, OR KIND ACT FOR THE DAY
_____
_____
_____
_____

We have a choice about how we take what happens to us in our life and whether or not we allow it to turn us.
- Angelina Jolie

blessed af

JAN FEB MAR APR MAY JUN JUL AUG SEP OCT NOV DEC
1 2 3 4 5 6 7 8 9 10 11 12 13 14 15 16 17 18 19 20 21 22 23 24 25 26 27 28 29 30 31

SOMETHING GOOD THAT HAPPENED TODAY

_____
_____
_____
_____

SOMEONE OR SOMETHING I AM THANKFUL FOR AND WHY

_____
_____
_____
_____

MY GOOD DEED, HAPPY THOUGHT, OR KIND ACT FOR THE DAY

_____
_____
_____
_____

Those who have the ability to be grateful are the ones who have the ability to achieve greatness.
- Steve Maraboli

blessed af

JAN FEB MAR APR MAY JUN JUL AUG SEP OCT NOV DEC
1 2 3 4 5 6 7 8 9 10 11 12 13 14 15 16 17 18 19 20 21 22 23 24 25 26 27 28 29 30 31

SOMETHING GOOD THAT HAPPENED TODAY
___
___
___
___

SOMEONE OR SOMETHING I AM THANKFUL FOR AND WHY
___
___
___
___

MY GOOD DEED, HAPPY THOUGHT, OR KIND ACT FOR THE DAY
___
___
___
___

Whatever you appreciate and give thanks for will increase in your life.
- Sanaya Roman

Made in the USA
Coppell, TX
27 July 2020